Dr. Michele Reed

The Fit Doc's Guide To Real Life, Real Fitness, Real Health

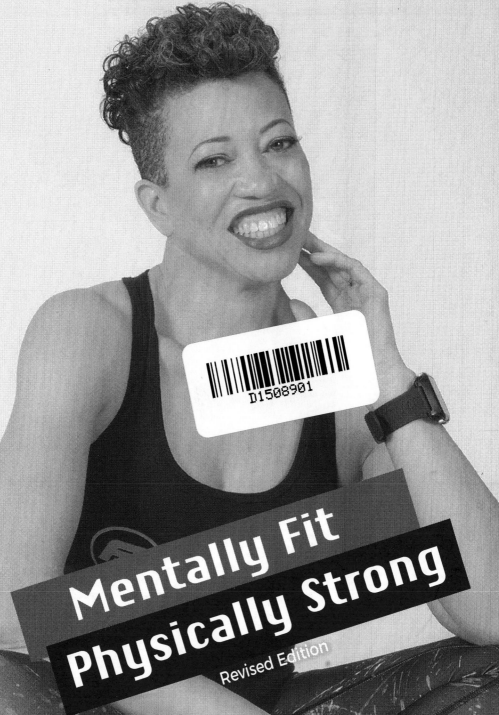

Mentally Fit Physically Strong

Revised Edition

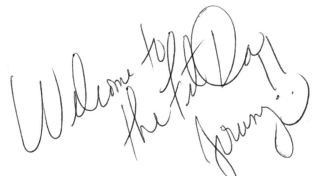

Mentally Fit Physically Strong

The Fit Doc's Guide To Real Life, Real Fitness, Real Health
Revised Edition

Dr. Michele Reed

Dr. Michele Reed is one of those special physicians who understands that good health begins with a mindset of fitness. In Mentally Fit, Physically Strong, Dr. Reed shares the elements of this mindset from her own life and from 20 years of serving patients. Through her accessible voice, Dr. Reed's writing compels and inspires us to get moving and embrace healthy living. Thank God for the gift of this book, and for the gift of Dr. Michele Reed.

Rev. Dr. Patrick G. Duggan, Pastor
Congregational Church of South Hempstead
United Church of Christ

Dr. Michele's book serves as an awesome reminder of the things I forget very often due to my hectic work schedule: health is just as much a priority as going to work. Eating healthy and working out is about lifestyle change not just losing inches and weight. It is about making time to put yourself first. As a friend of Dr. Michele, I am elated to be a part of this journey with her and strongly encourage other women to get healthy with us!

Loni Love
Comedian and Talk Show Host

The "R" in Reed stands for Real! Dr. Michele Reed is real in her commitment to living a healthy lifestyle and also inspiring others to do the same. She is real in that she not only "talks the talk," but also "walks the walk" and "runs the race." I am real glad that she started me on the journey.

Wilma Holmes Tootle
Lifelong Mentor

My mother said, "You can have everything - just not all at once." Then I met Dr. Reed, a mother, wife, doctor, business owner, and marathoner to name a few. She has learned the formula for having it all, at once, without losing your mind. There are plenty of 'superwomen' who are clearly juggling more than they should. Mentally Fit, Physically Strong teaches us how to not only navigate life's terrain, but to thrive and truly enjoy the process. This isn't a book for someone looking for a magic pill to make life go smoothly. Dr. Reed encourages us to first step up and be proactive about our health and fitness. She imparts bitesize portions of wisdom for sustainable change. I've watched her live by these principles. Those who have followed her lead go from frazzled superwomen to being grounded and confident in their ability to take on life's next adventure.

Angelique Perrin
Syndicated Radio Personality

There are major benefits to the real life integration of self, health, family, and work for optimal wellness. The Fit Doc inspires real people to prioritize and experience success at improving and maintaining a healthy lifestyle. She envisions a world where individuals take charge and stamp out at-risk behaviors, own their health, and live their best life. Practical, motivating, and engaging, The Fit Doc encourages readers to take small steps to make a huge difference in overall wellness.

Larthenia Howard, Ed.D.
Author of *Challenging Mediocrity*

Mentally Fit, Physically Strong: The Fit Doc's Guide to Real Life, Real Fitness, Real Health Revised Edition

Copyright © 2018 by Michele C. Reed

All rights reserved. Published in the United States by Pipe Publishing, a division of the Stimuknowlogy Institute LLC Fort Pierce, Florida.

www.writeabookin31days.com

Mentally Fit, Physically Strong may be purchased in bulk for educational, business, or promotional use. For information please contact **DrMichele@FitDoc.com**

Library of Congress Cataloging-In-Publication Data Reed, Michele C.

Mentally Fit, Physically Strong: the fit doc's guide to real life, real fitness, real health/Michele C. Reed

-Revised Edition.

ISBN 978-0-9844475-8-9

Health, Fitness & Dieting   2. Psychology & Counseling

Library of Congress Control Number: 2017952969

Cover and interior design by Stacey Grainger
Cover photo and concept design by Tricia Messeroux

Printed in the United States of America
Revised Edition

Dedication

To my wonderful husband, Walter Scott Kershaw, our sons Marcus and Stephen, and my family.

Thank you for your enduring support and patience. Without you, this project would not have been achieved. Because of you, I show up better and healthier to serve the world.

Contents

Foreword

Dr. Michele C. Reed reminds us that health is not measured, or assured, by the absence of disease. She encourages us to secure health through the adoption of specific personal behaviors and lifestyle strategies.

Dr. Reed shares her personal journey to achieving 'mental and physical health' with the readers through stories and advice. This Fit Doc is not just a role model. She provides a roadmap with (frequent) cautionary warnings that achieving health cannot be passively accomplished. Dr. Reed emphasizes, throughout this wonderful book, that being healthy is an active and individualized process that requires personal focus, commitment, attitude, and sustained work. Dr. Michele Reed's career in medicine is, and has been, an example of a sustained commitment to community and population health that we, in academic medicine, aspire to achieve in all of our NYITCOM students and alumni. As a black female physician, she represents the power of diversity and the importance of including diverse perspectives in the delivery of quality health and preventive care. I consider myself a privileged witness to who Dr. Reed is and the professional that she has become.

Barbara Ross-Lee, DO, FACOFP
New York Institute of Technology
Vice President Health Sciences and Medical Affairs
Executive Director of the AACOM Health Policy Fellowship
National Osteopathic Medical Association,
Co-founder and Member Board of Trustees

Introduction

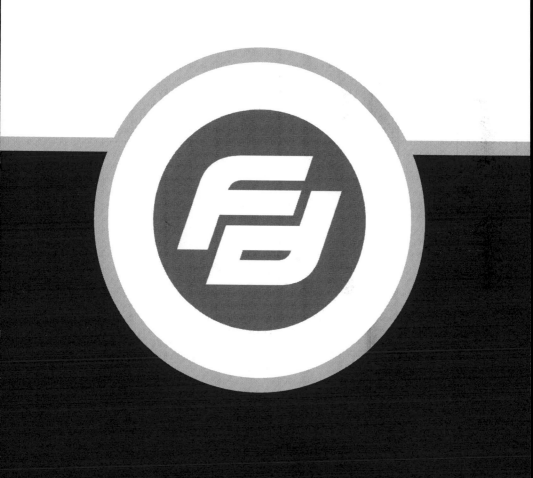

Introduction

The Making of "Fit Doc"

For an overwhelming number of people, there is a belief that the actors seen on TV "have it all together." I want to set the tone straight before we begin this journey together by saying, "I am not superwoman!" I am a regular person just like you, with my own beauty and blemishes. Far too often we believe what we want is not possible. We believe our lives are fixed and we cannot control our destinies. I will admit, my life is hurried at times and I feel as if balance, or harmony, is an elusive target. In this increasingly fast paced world, finding time to catch your breath and relax is difficult, let alone time to consider a plan for a healthy lifestyle. This book is not about a complicated set of exercise routines, or overcomplicating your life with a million things to do. My goal is to challenge your belief systems, shatter un-resourceful thoughts and behaviors, and guide you into creating better habits that will lead to a healthier lifestyle, both mentally and physically. As a result, I hope to help you make better choices with the foods you eat, uncover hidden motivations behind exercise, and identify reasons you want a better you.

You might be thinking to yourself:

- I work 90 plus hours a week. When do you want me to work out?

- I would work out more if I did not have this hairstyle or did not sweat so much.

- Gym memberships cost a lot and my funds are already tapped to the max.

- Eating healthy requires more time to prepare. With a family to feed, I do not have time for all of that.

No matter how overwhelmed life may seem, we all, ultimately, have a responsibility to take care of our health. It is a matter of choice. You can choose to practice unhealthy habits or choose to practice habits that render better health. The commitment you make with yourself, for yourself, is one of the most important decisions you can make. Most of us would agree that the benefits of health and wellness far outweigh the challenges. With proper goal setting and a plan of accountability, I believe a healthy lifestyle is attainable.

As a physician, I have been on this grind for almost twenty years, helping patients, and the communities I serve live healthier lifestyles. My philosophy on healthy living comes from a number of experiences that I will personally share with you throughout this book. Prior to the start of this journey, it became apparent that there was a clear disconnect between my patient's perceptions of what it meant to have a healthy lifestyle, and the research that supported overall health and wellness. I noticed an alarming trend throughout threads of conversations; there was this notion that good health was purely contingent on DNA, or only achievable if a person is wealthy.

This thought process was real for so many of my patients. The definition of healthy habits seemed obscure and was totally off the mark in some cases. One of my patients believed eating shrimp fried rice everyday was healthier than eating chicken or pork fried rice, simply because it feels lighter on the stomach. Unbeknownst to her, she was sending her cholesterol levels through the roof and putting herself at a greater risk for a stroke or heart attack. Still, a great number of patients resolved to accept their temporary conditions and ailments as permanent. It would seem as if little or nothing could be done to resolve their present existence.

Many of the new patients came to me for a prescription, rather than preventive counseling or treatment. A paradigm shift had to occur. I felt confused and was disheartened by the unhealthy mindsets of my patients. At the same time, I became more and more dissatisfied with my own health profile. I ran and exercised, but I needed to do more to keep myself engaged. Oftentimes our hearts are in the right place when attempting to achieve a goal. However, if we are not totally committed to the process and the follow through, we risk reverting to old habits that are counterproductive. Fitting into a smaller dress for that twentieth year high school reunion may not be inspiring enough to get you to LA Fitness every morning for circuit training. On a personal level, you might want to look your best for the peers who knew you in the eleventh grade, but if you are not connected to the process, you will default to unhealthy routines.

Like so many of my patients, I was operating in default, and needed a change. Quickly.

Sometime after having a heart to heart with myself about my own need to change some of my health habits, I witnessed the most inspiring thing. During Sunday brunch with my husband (one of my favorite pastimes), I noticed women from all over the country flocking into the lobby of the Long Island Marriott. The majority of them were wearing tutus, tiaras, and boas while carrying a single red rose. They had just completed either a 5K or Half Marathon. I guess I was so intrigued by it because my preconceived notions about the "ideal runner" were shattered. In my mind running, on that level, was a sport that attracted only thin, slender women. But these women looked like me! They were tall, short, full-figured, slim you name it. Before I realized it, I was thinking out loud, "I would love to do that." It was in that moment that my earth shifted. My love affair with running revived just like that.

Inspired by what I had witnessed, I continued to run on my own for some time. Then I remembered one of the ladies in the lobby was wearing a t-shirt with the words, "Black Girls Run" inscribed across the front. One of my patients had told me about the group, but up to that point I had not bothered to find out more. Upon further investigation of the group I came across the organization's vision statement:

"We aspire to take a comprehensive and creative approach to improve the health statistics of women of color."

BLACK GIRLS RUN VISION

This truly resonated within my soul. The organization was in full alignment with my healthy lifestyle goals as a health professional, wife, mother, and an athlete. Black Girls Run was on a mission and was dedicated to helping Black women (just like me) on their quest to healthy living. Through the process of self-awareness, the pieces came together and I was off and running towards a new lifestyle. This was exactly what I needed - a supportive and nurturing group of like-minded people to help me reach my goals. Fast forward three years, I am a few pounds lighter, a few dress sizes smaller, and I have run two world major marathons – the New York City Marathon and the Chicago Marathon.

But that is not the real story. Along my personal journey to better health, I met some of the most amazing people. My life has certainly been enhanced and my ability to help my patients has changed for the better. Not only do I continue to improve my health, but have also increased my capacity to affect desired change in others. By sharing my experiences, others are inspired to set goals for healthier lifestyle changes. My sphere of influence has allowed me to help people like Dionne, a member of Black Girls Run and Merrick Bicycle Tri Team, who is also one of my patients. She came to my office with a very high cholesterol level, and sought advice on the next logical move to improve her health. After an examination, I offered her two options: she could begin medication to lower her cholesterol, or she could begin to make healthier changes to her lifestyle. It did not take her long to make a decision, especially considering the possibility of taking medication for the rest of her life. We immediately started a conversation around lifestyle changes that could make a big difference, not just in her cholesterol numbers, but in her overall wellbeing. To date, Dionne is healthy and she makes decisions regarding life choices in different ways. She went from running as purely a form of exercise, to becoming a triathlete and participating in Ironman competitions. My impact on Dionne and others led to the brand "Fit Doc," a name I was affectionately given by my Black Girls Run team. The name has stuck like glue. The more I consider the health epidemic of our nation and the unhealthy habits of those I see on a daily basis, the more I become committed to live up to the meaning of "Fit Doc" to the absolute best of my ability.

The *Fit Doc's Guide* is designed to be used as support as you begin and continue to tweak your overall health and wellness regiment. It is not a substitute for routine doctor visits, or information and medical advice you have received from your personal health care provider. Each chapter is a short discussion, in practical and easy to follow language, of topics that have supported my wellness goals the most. After each discussion, I offer several tips for you to consider on your journey to experiencing life at its peak. There is space below each tip for you to jot notes and thoughts. By the end of the book, hopefully you will have developed a personal plan of action that you can commit to and continue to monitor, and one that you can share with your health care provider as a sign of your dedication to wellness. Be open to sharing your authentic self on this journey. It takes work on all levels to change yourself into the person you want to become. Rate the degree to which you are or are not applying different practices. My ultimate desire is that you seriously ponder where you are physically and mentally and make adjustments as necessary.

So, as I mentioned earlier, I am not a superwoman. I am not the fastest, I am not the strongest, but I am in the best shape of my life. I am setting personal bests and personal records along life's amazing race. I am a real physician, providing real medicine, living a really full and productive life. I invite you to come and run with me, "Fit Doc," in the race for better health and a more optimized life. You can do it! I am a living testimony and so are you!

CHAPTER ONE
The Starting Line

"I'm always nervous.
If I wasn't nervous, it would be weird.
I get the same feeling at all the big
races. It's part of the routine,
and I accept it.
It means I'm there and I'm ready."

ALLYSON FELIX

Unknown Territory

For many people, the starting line has always seemed like a leap into the unknown. The range of emotions cycling through the body during this time can cause many people to either not start the race, or to run it poorly. As a runner since elementary school, I have always been challenged, mentally, at the starting line. Questions in my head would toss about feverishly.

- Did I train hard enough?

- Will I get tired and be able to finish?

- How will I run this race? Should I be aggressive or passive?

- Will I win or lose?

As I approach the start of any journey in my life, I, like others in similar situations, am unsure of the outcomes. This feeling of uncertainty is normal. It is a sign that you are aware and present in the moment. This inner dialogue might seem like noise in a place where you need to be calm, but it is only a reminder to focus solely on the goal at hand.

The starting line is a lonely place at times. The "oomph" that you have when you first set out to change your life will flicker. Smiles that once lit up your face at the thought of you eating right and exercising consistently will be flipped upside down every now and then. And, there will be many times when you may feel as if you are in this race by yourself.

You Are.

The Reset I Needed

After giving birth to my twin boys, it was hard to shake off some of the excess weight from the pregnancy. Although I had immediately started to train by running and biking, I was not losing

3

the weight like I wanted. This was one of the most frustrating experiences for me to date. However, I was not in it alone. Several of my patients were experiencing similar frustrations. You know it is bad when you and your patients are not eating for health benefits. During this same time, I was working long hours at the practice and it completely threw me off my eating and sleeping schedule. Sometimes, I would not leave the office until 10:30 p.m. or later. My husband, Scott and I would eat dinner late at nights and then go straight home and hit the bed. Not the recipe for healthy living right? I needed help!

Implementing just a few of the changes I found during my research, I was able to make a lot of progress. My regular routine seemed as if it had been supercharged. The results were amazing to say the least. I cannot tell you how many times I have heard, "Oh my God, you're losing so much weight," or "You're so skinny. This can't be healthy." I will be the first to admit, it was hard to ignore some of the talk, especially coming from friends who knew my mission. But, instead of taking it personally, or getting offended, I used the comments as fuel and feedback. It gave me fuel to keep going

4

because I was receiving the benefits of my new lifestyle plan, and feedback to increase muscle toning for an even healthier look.

The journey seemed lonely at times, but I knew I was on the right track. The results were all the proof I needed. Family and friends meant well in their responses to my changes. They continued to encourage me, but the truth is, I was on the road to self-improvement alone. No one else around me was altering their lifestyle or eating habits. Nope. I was in it alone. The journey was mine, and I had to own the process for myself.

Inspiration for Change

I shared a snippet of my lifestyle challenge and change to encourage you at the starting line. Similar to my experience, you may start solo – just you and your goal. There is a lot of value at this stage. This is the opportunity for you to get crystal clear about your goals, dreams, hopes, and desires. What is it, exactly, that you want for yourself? Alone, you can quietly reflect and converse with yourself. Ask yourself, "In all honesty, am I doing the best I can to be the healthiest version of myself?" Sit still and wait for the response. I have a sneaky suspicion that intuition will nudge you to consider the areas in your life where change would result in an even better you.

Relationships Play a Key Role

Sometimes even the smallest adjustment can make the biggest difference. In my quest, one of the changes that really paid off was in altering the way I interacted with close companions. Although I started solo, I eventually wanted to connect with others who had an interest in better health. As relational beings, connecting is very important in obtaining overall wellbeing. If you are aspiring to become a better teacher, it might be wise to surround yourself with other educators. It does not mean that you will not hang out with your friends who are not educators, but the interaction within the relationship may shift as a result of your newfound goals.

If you are concerned about being the "funny acting friend" to some people, do not worry. This race is about YOU. The people who care about you will understand. I interject here because I had to change the way I interacted with my friends and be aware of the challenges in many cases. If I was going to embrace this new healthy way of living, I could not be at a happy hour indulging in 2-for-1 appetizers every week with my girls. I am not saying that I will never grab a hot wing or two, but I am more conscious and mindful of how I spend my time and the choices I make concerning my health.

With this new goal of mine, I started to suggest that we engage in more physical activities such as running, or any type of physical activity that would make us sweat, instead of always meeting up to eat and socialize. Some friends came along for the ride and some did not. Ultimately, I made the necessary changes to support my goals, and managed to enlist a few supporters along the way, who are happier and healthier because of the shifts we made together.

Discover the Vision – Set a Goal

The point of all of this is, the race is a personal quest for your freedom. It may require a lot of mental toughness and fortitude but you must be vision oriented in order to stick through the tough times. Having a goal in mind when beginning any process is critical. Without a predetermined destination, you are open to arriving anywhere, thereby exacerbating dissatisfaction. I challenged myself to eat healthy, and set daily goals to achieving it. This included a progress tracker and weekly check-in with my accountability partner for motivation, and a reminder of my 'big picture vision' for both health and wellness. My random workouts turned into a more crystal clear, focused, and attainable game plan for success. This preparation at the starting line helped me to conquer bigger goals like the New York City and Chicago Marathons.

Identify Your Support Systems

Support is always readily available when you're taking steps in the right direction. My neighbor, Cheryl, soon became my 5:45 a.m. running buddy. I am thankful for her support during the mornings when it was tough to get up and face the brisk morning air. Cheryl and I also joined other members of Black Girls Run on weekly running outings. This helped support my goals immensely. Throughout the process of training for the marathon, which is one of the most daring feats for an individual, I also became a source of inspiration and strength for other women. Just as much I helped them, their presence kept me lifted throughout the process.

It is not easy lacing up your sneakers at 6 a.m. when everyone else is getting zzz's. It takes a special level of dedication and self-care to push past moments when you don't have a crew of cheerleaders to root for you. Your race in life, like my runs, is personal. Others may act as a source of support, but they cannot run for you!

Family, Friends, and Sometimes Foes

I am reminded of one of my colleagues who wanted to shed some weight. She started to cook with fresh vegetables, less sugar and salt, and she added exercise to her routine. Her health goal to shed pounds and change her lifestyle sounded like the right thing to do. However, her efforts were met with great resistance when she prepared healthy meals for her husband. Changes in the food preparation did not sit well with him. He wanted the same sodium laced, high fructose infused dishes he had grown to love.

Resistance. Tension. Friction

The sooner you grasp the idea that those around you simply play a role in your race but are not the race itself, the better off you will be. On your journey, some people will serve in roles as coaches, distractors, and cheerleaders, and some will be of no consequence. My charge to you is to remain undaunted. Keep your eyes on the prize!

After a long conversation with one of my patients, she agreed it was time to seriously take better care of herself. She had been facing prediabetes and more complicated health issues from the year before. Changes were not optional if she wanted to experience health and longevity. She needed to work on changing her eating habits and start an exercise routine, immediately. Heeding my advice, her efforts were noticeable and her commitment was obvious. She reported feeling better and having the necessary energy to get through long days at work. Although it was clear that her changes were for the better, the moment she started to shed weight, her close friend told her to find a new doctor because she looked so "unhealthy." As she shared this with me, I reminded her not everyone is going to be at her starting line with her, but she should keep doing what is best for her anyway. Thank goodness, for the sake of her health, she followed through and has been able to maintain a healthy weight since following through on her plan of action. Because of her perseverance, her friend has now become my patient and the two support one another in an exercise regiment. Imagine if she had not made a sincere commitment at her starting line.

As you travel through life and experience positioning at the starting line, you may look around and notice you are the only person there. You might feel alone. But again, here is where you have one of the greatest opportunities to see the person you want to become. In that moment, choose to bring her along as your ride or die friend.

Start Well and Finish Strong

Each year I construct a vision board and determine a new starting line for moving through the different areas of my life. I review personal, health and professional goals. I consider my closest relationships, those with my husband, sons, family, and friends. In the professional corner, I consider risks and how to make gains in the upcoming year. I list particular scriptures to guide my intentions. On a personal level, I hone in on physical and mental areas for improvement. My vision board serves as the guiding light for how I'll start my new year. These reminders help guide me on a journey towards rewards and greatness.

The goal is to start well and finish strong. A clear focus on what you want, combined with a dedicated plan of action, will help you achieve any type of goal you set. Remember, there will be noise, the road might be lonely, but a personal vision that compels deliberate action is able to confront any challenge.

I'll see you at the Starting Line.

Fit Doc Checkup

» Do you see yourself in the same place you were last year, or are you at a different Starting Line? What can you do to impact a greater difference?

» The Starting Line presents an inner dialogue that can be filled with a range of emotions: fear, excitement, anxiety, uncertainty etc. What emotions do you have running through your head when you are at the beginning of a life change or very big decision? How do your emotions influence your behaviors?

» When you set goals, you are literally planting a seed. Planting requires digging. Dig deep within to decide what truly matters most to you. Prioritize ideas, projects, and action plans. Indicate what moves will get you closer to your goals.

» Eliminate the weeds as soon as they are recognized.

» Learn to truly relax. When you go through change and unwelcomed times in life, relax and get comfortable with the idea of different. In most cases, different is different. It is not better or worse, just different. Rest in the comfort of change and different. A conditioned body and mind is necessary. Identify an area in your life where change is necessary. What actions can you take to embrace this change?

» Declare selfishness as an asset. This is selfishness in a healthy way. As we learn from air travel, it is advisable to place on your oxygen mask first so you are better able to help others. A healthy form of selfishness relates to attending to your needs so you are prepared to take care of the needs of others. What outside influences do you see as potential challenges to your new lease on self-care?

NOTES

NOTES

CHAPTER TWO
Breaking the Wall

Your internal conversation begins the initiation towards any external change.

We All Face the Moment at Some Point

We all know life does not always flow as smoothly as we would like. You will find a good rhythm that works for you and out of nowhere, life will throw you a curveball. Heck, it might even throw you several curveballs and you will manage to dodge one only to get hit by four others. Life has a way of taking you off course, and, if you're not careful, you can become discouraged. As much as we believe strong bones and muscles power us through tough situations, the mind serves as the true engine behind every action.

When we have been knocked off our envisioned path, the one we seek diligently, we tend to get discouraged. The energy built up over time suddenly hits a wall. All the progress and excitement rushes out and it is easy to come to a complete halt. Hitting the wall is usually a term that is reserved for athletes to explain when energy stored in the muscles suddenly vanishes. However, people also encounter these moments in real life situations. Once you have hit the proverbial wall, you soon realize it is your mind that has actually done the checking out, and not your physical body.

Time and time again, when I have hit the wall of life, I reached for resources that have served me well.

> "I am stronger than I think I am."

An affirmation of inner strength can turn a temporary setback into momentum for a breakthrough. When I need encouragement to keep going, I simply repeat, *"I am stronger than I think I am."* This mantra represents courage and perseverance that I tap into to move me through, and over the finish lines. While doing planks, I recite it aloud when my core feels weak. I recite it in my head when I feel challenged by difficult conversations with patients about their health. I recite it when my lovely twin sons challenge every nerve in my body. There is no doubt, my daily successes are determined by the quality of my thoughts and belief system. A mantra gives life to beliefs.

Connections are Everywhere

For me, health and wellness are connected to everything. With respect to this belief, I am charged with engaging in the necessary activities that will keep my physical, mental, and spiritual self on a level that is poised for continual and healthy growth.

I know eating donuts, cookies, and cakes raise my blood sugar level and increase my chance of diabetes.

- *I know living a sedentary lifestyle adds inches to every undesirable place on my body.*

I know a funky attitude attracts negative people and situations, which disrupt my inner peace.

Each morning I set intentions for the day. I speak about positive things I want to see manifested in my life. As a wife, I think about ways to be a better partner, listener, and supporter of my husband, Scott. In my role as a mother, I want to be a nurturer, a source of inspiration, and a safe space for my two growing young men. I am also responsible for guiding the health and wellness of every single patient who walks into my office. Because I am a part of the process for my patients living long and healthy lives, I speak wisdom, patience, and success into my spirit. In a vigil to break the wall of lethargy, my day includes a healthy workout routine that may consist of running, light weights, or a quick ride on my bike. A healthy breakfast of proper nutrition supports sustained energy throughout the day and helps to maintain mental clarity until bedtime.

As I stated at the start of this conversation, life can often seem complicated. We are confronted with obstacles, performing daily obligations, and constantly juggling responsibilities. Although the routine, my personal support systems, may appear unrealistic to some, it is as a result of a habit I formed and took repeated practice to master. Hopefully, you will consider a plan of action that can be built into your lifestyle – one that motivates and infuses freshness.

Running Through the Wall

A valuable source of validation can be found in a gentle reminder of the greatness you both possess and seek as you make efforts to push through tough times. In a desire to help break the cycle of "hitting the wall", here is an exercise I use when attempting to facilitate change in my health and wellness coaching clients: follow the process of developing a personal mantra that will empower and offer insight.

The first part of developing a mantra requires recall and reflection on your top five accomplishments over the past year. You may have landed a new job or secured a promotion, shed unwanted pounds or established healthier eating habits, or forgiven someone whom you had resented because of an offense. Take some time to consider accomplishments you are most proud to note.

Next, make a list of the steps you took in order to achieve success. Do this for each of the five accomplishments. One or two sentences is sufficient in this step.

Step three is to explain why the accomplishment is of value to you.

The final step of part one is to summarize your statements into a powerful affirmation, or what I refer to as a *wall breaker*.

Example:

Accomplishment: I traveled to five new countries this past year.

Steps:

Set a goal to travel, noting possible sacrifices.

- Did research (culture, funds needed) for each trip I wanted to take.

- Included dates for travel on calendar.

- Created a budget that identified funds for travel/leisure.

- Instead of buying things, I invested in experiences.

Value: Travel adds value to my life and happiness.

Wall Breaker: "I am committed to traveling because it provides happiness and adds value to my life."

Part two of this process asks you to follow the above steps while you recall and reflect on five shortcomings or disappointments that impacted you in the past year. Once you have completed each step, summarize a *wall breaker* that encourages you to shift motivation towards accomplishment.

24

Example:

Shortcoming/Disappointment: I gained 30 pounds this past year.

Steps:

Set a goal in my mind, but did not write it down.

- Inconsistent in monitoring weight regularly.
- Did not follow the original meal plan, or prep foods.
- Inconsistent in exercise.
- Auto-pilot eating.
- Ate out more often than a home prepared meal.

Value: Health and wellness are important so I am at my best for the grandchildren.

Wall Breaker: "I prep meals consistently so my weight and health are optimal."

Once this activity is complete, write each wall breaker, or mantra, on a separate index card. I typically use different colors and employ creativity when noting wall breakers. Some of my clients punch holes in the top left corner of each card and secure them on a key ring. Others have taped them inside their cars, or onto their bathroom mirrors. I know several persons who carry the wall breaker cards in their purses or portfolios. No matter where you choose to place the cards, the idea is to keep them in a place where you constantly see them and can be reminded to review them- repeating each at least twice a day. As you create a habit of reviewing each summary, and as you begin to memorize them, the wall breakers will serve as a tool to unlocking the person you know you can be. Tap into the awesome power of your own personal conviction. Remember, a mere recital of wall breakers is nothing without action. Make a commitment to "do" what you "say."

Align Internal to the External

Your internal conversation begins the initiation towards any external change. True change happens when you are in tune with your belief system and act accordingly. As a runner, I often get compliments or comments about my appearance. This may be partly because I am almost always wearing my favorite red lipstick. Wearing lipstick is awesome and certainly brightens my mood, but I make it a habit to check the congruency between my mind (mental wellness) and my body (outside appearance). As a society, we are constantly encouraged to focus on the outside—the physical being or the attire. Sometimes we may wear makeup to mask the ugliness we feel inside, and to appear more beautiful on the outside. I make it a conscientious practice to double check because whatever I choose to mask on the inside will eventually show all over. I make it my duty to nurture my mental faculties by reciting wall breakers, exercising, and eating foods essential to my health. A healthy spirit and mind is as important as a healthy body.

In my practice, I often see patients who have the outer appearance together, but are in the worse shape of their life. They are busy 'looking good' to the visible eye, yet have "hit the wall" when it comes to practicing healthy habits. It becomes a regular routine to forget medications that combat blood pressure or diabetes, and blow off one exercise routine after the other. I sometimes inquire, "You look good, but are you feeling good?" My interaction with patients extend beyond the surface of a usual doctor-patient relationship. I want to know about their stressors, their worries,

27

and their internal challenges because they are the mental blocks that cause them to hit the wall and obstruct their absolute best. Physical health is important to me, but I am dually concerned with my clients' mental well-being. It is all related. When you feel good on the inside, you are liberated to do amazing things with your life - which translates to your outer appearance.

> Mascara only masks, but if you take on the task of developing healthier habits you'll grow fast, and last.

The Journey Begins with the Start

Starting a new lifestyle change is not for the weak of heart. It takes a strong person to realize they need to make a change, and be willing to march to the *starting line* of change.

It is encouraging when you move in the right direction and the universe aligns in your favor. Roadblocks will begin to move once you decide to start. Resources show up and people are motivated to help you along the journey. When forging a new path, or habit, there is strength in numbers, but initiation of the first step is the key.

I have met some of the most amazing and unlikely exercise partners on my journey to health and wholeness. During my sons' basketball tournament, I wore a "Black Girls Run" t-shirt. A woman named Tia approached me and expressed that she liked my shirt. The more we talked, the more we realized our commonalities. I talked to her about the organization and we decided to run together. Since that initial meeting, we've traveled together and she also helped me train for the New York City Marathon.

You meet people in the most unlikely places in your pursuit of passion. The universe conspires to put the right people in your path to motivate you and challenge you to greater heights. My friend from church, Ashleigh, is another one of those people. Although she was already running solo, through a chance meeting, she joined my other running partner, Shari and I, in becoming members of Black Girls Run. The signs are truly everywhere when you are on the right path. You simply have to be open to the possibilities of change. Synergy amongst Ashleigh, Tia and me was greater than the energy I had alone. I realized it took a collective energy to build something great. My neighbor, Ryon, is always ready for a bike ride anytime of the day and has even ventured out on some early morning long runs to chaperone me and my friends. So, although the journey is personal and lonely at times, I found strength through networks of support.

One of the best support networks for me, aside from my friends, is my husband. When I was training for the NYC TCS Marathon, Scott would leave the house with me at 3 a.m. so I could do my 18 - 22 miles runs before my office hours. He rode his bike, tailing me on each mile. It was comforting to know that I had a support system right at home. This partnership has been awesome! On the days of my runs, he exercised as well. My personal journey inspired him. A double win!

Fit Doc Checkup

» What belief system do you have that potentially hinders your success?

» Take a few moments to contemplate the origin of your belief systems. From whom, or where, did you get beliefs about health, career, wealth, Spirit? How do these beliefs show up for you today?

» When has there been a wall that you could not seem to evade? What made you feel as if you couldn't push forward and continue along the path?

» What could you have done differently?

» The universe is always conspiring for your good. Think of instances when good things have shown up as affirmation that you were on the right path.

» The human will is strong, but at times we get weak and jaded from the mission. When your spirit needs a lift, where or who do you turn to for strength?

NOTES

CHAPTER THREE
It's All in the Stride: Reasons Why You Can

The world we've grown accustomed to, is changing by the second and at our fingertips.

Microwaveable.

Quick.

Painless.

Change is a Process

The demand to get faster, more efficient, and better is present in just about every aspect of life. You feel the pressure of the supervisor's pushy demands when he or she sends a snippy email about a project that was just assigned an hour ago. Your children's elementary school is pushing him or her to be college-ready before they've set foot into the sixth grade. Need groceries? Don't worry about dressing and hopping into your car - there is an app for that. We are in the NOW generation. The immediacy of our needs today is setting the tone for how the future will evolve. In a world where "I Love You" can now be dumbed down to an emoji, it is imperative that we constantly work to remain true to fundamentals that will stand the test of time.

You can run from the real work of change, only to eventually realize "quick" just does not cut it if authentic sustainability is the goal. We know exercise is important, yet seem to come up with millions of reasons as to why it is not a priority. It is common for someone to say to me, "Dr. Reed, I have no energy. Can you write a prescription for weight loss pills? I need to lose weight before I start to exercise."

What I hear is...

"Dr. Reed, I want to lose weight now and do it with little to no effort."

The reality is, weight may not be the culprit of low energy. I know many full-figured women who have loads of energy, and thin women who have zero to no energy. Admittedly, I have had many patients make the same request. To put it bluntly, they want a new body immediately. Like yesterday. They seem desperate for a change. I say desperate although not many of them wanted to work at a change in habits, or a change in mindset. As discussed in the previous chapter, change begins in the mind. In this scenario, a pill represents an immediate fix, a microwaveable solution to a process that naturally takes time. While I empathize with the need to feel healthier ASAP, I also want to charge patients to begin doing the work it takes to get the body they deserve.

I think it would be safe to say that most people love the results of working out. Who would not like to comfortably fit into clothes of a desired size? Do you know anyone who does not love a nice compliment? In obtaining a healthy body and image, we must fall in love with the process just as much as the promise. The degree to which you embrace each step in the journey determines your measure of success. Without a solution oriented approach, you'll likely find yourself "hitting the wall" over and over, looking for shortcuts or an easy fix. The attitude of "*now, now, now!*" has to be destroyed in order to get the results we want for the long haul. Oftentimes our mindsets are crippling the energy needed to win the race of life. We approach a marathon with a sprinter's mentality and therefore lose the race. In my daily life, I encounter women who think of every imaginable excuse to avoid doing what is best for their health. I have heard everything from not having enough time for exercise, to healthy food costs too much. Let me pause for a moment to dispel several myths.

Myth Busters with Dr. Michele

@MrsNoTiempo:

I don't have enough time to work out. By the time I get home after working 8 hours and preparing dinner for my family, it's time for me to go to bed again. Where do I fit in working out with such a busy schedule?

@AskDrMichele:

Most people believe they need to be in the gym for long periods of time to warrant the term "workout." In fact, studies show that thirty minutes of exercise can help trigger the 'feel good' hormones, endorphins, in the brain. These endorphins help create a sense of euphoria in the body, which emits more energy, reduces stress, and aids in better sleep. Overall, most people feel better. Cardio exercises such as walking, running, jumping rope, basketball, boxing, and other exercises that increase the heart rate are great for thirty minutes of fun. This thirty minutes set aside each day is for you and your health. Prioritize your health the same way you prioritize paying bills or watching your favorite sitcom. It is challenging to obtain and maintain health and wellness without a semblance of dedicated physical activity. Under the supervision of your physician, try thirty minutes of exercise in some form for five days and then gauge how you feel. Most who do notice an improvement in mood, clothes fit more comfortably, and energy increases. It is important to start. Monitor how you feel and decide if self-improvement is worth the effort.

@HairdoBoo313:

My job will fire me in a heartbeat if I walk in with my hair all sweated out and I'm looking tired. I am a heavy sweater. How am I supposed to exercise and maintain the do?

@AskDr.Michele:

I am in the same boat as you. I have a job where employees and patients will look at me like I am crazy if I report to work looking rough and rugged. But here is the deal. I exercise four times per week. Workouts are scheduled around my hair appointments. I usually visit the hair salon once a week on Tuesday mornings. I exercise Monday, Tuesday, Saturday, and Sunday mornings. When my hair does not look the best, I sometimes compensate by wearing a head cap or using gel to slick my hair back. If you cannot sport a hat to the office, maybe try a ponytail, high or low bun, or a headband until you see your hair stylist. Several of my patients have chosen to go natural. They find it easier to maintain their natural hair while adapting to a new lifestyle. It costs to maintain beauty. Invest in your overall health, both your inner and outer beauty.

@Motherof4Kids:

My husband and I have staggered schedules. When I'm at work he's at home, and vice versa. The majority of the child rearing responsibilities rest on me. Whenever I try to work out, kids - ages 11, 7, and 5- pull me in every direction. They're a hyperactive bunch, so I have to keep my eyes on them at all times.

@AskDrMichele:

Believe it or not, it sounds like you have the perfect situation. You have three energetic kids who need something to do. Have you ever thought about having family fitness nights? My family enjoys running a lot, so we go on runs through the park together. It is a great way to bond and at the same time, accomplish my fitness goals. Kids are full of energy and love competition. I would strongly suggest creating a monthly calendar of group activities that you can do with them, and develop a healthy lifestyle together. Choose one or two nights out of the week and make it an evening of family wellness. Pack a few healthy snacks and soon your kids will be asking, "When are we having fitness night again?" Also, you might want to talk with your kids about personal health goals. Simplify the discussion in terms they will understand. Your consistency and intentionality will help create advocates and allies for healthy living.

Exercise and physical activity can have a positive effect on your everyday life. Even if you think you are too old or too out of shape to exercise, activity usually leads to more energy and improved health. If you are already active, keep up the good work and consider increasing or altering the intensity of workouts. If you do not exercise now, it is not too late to start. There are twenty four hours in a day. How will you prioritize your health and happiness?

Strut Your Stuff

University College London (UCL), in 2009, revealed it takes an average of sixty-six days to create a habit. I know, this is vastly different from what you may have heard. When most of us are asked the question, how many days does it take to form a habit, our response is likely the number twenty-one or thirty. According to UCL researchers, sixty-six is an average. Some of the participants in the study created a habit in less than that number of days, and for some, it was even longer. Regardless of the contested number, the bottom line is this—an optimally healthy body is one that moves and takes time to realize

Consider for a moment how much movement, do you participate in each week that is geared towards your health? If you already have a regular routine, do you track your progress so that you are aware of when it is time to shake up the usual regiment? In either situation, there are several benefits to integrating exercise into an intended healthy lifestyle that will later develop into a habit. It:

- Extends endurance and builds strength

- Burns calories

- Revs-up metabolism, even when body is at rest

- *Contours the body's physique*

- *Increases the flow of blood and stimulates the surface of the skin*

- *Promotes cardio-vascular wellness*

- *Increases and sustains energy*

After an intense workout, the body uses fuel from carbohydrates and glucose to help burn excess fat. This is especially insightful for anyone who desires to rid the body of unhealthy fat. Always remember, as little as thirty minutes of intense movement per day can increase the metabolism and shift your body into a fat burning machine. Shedding the excuses can definitely help shed the pounds.

Fit Doc Checkup

» *Examine your life for microwave, or quick fix, expectations. How do they inhibit you from embracing the process and ultimately growing as an individual?*

» *What are current or potential obstacles you may face when implementation a new outlook on health?*

» *Obstacles may be anything from resources, time, lack of family support etc.*

» *Take a moment to engage with me. Draft a question in the space below. Tweet to @AskDrMichele. Use the hashtag #FITDOC.*

» Mental and physical health are important to wellness. List several fun activities you can do with members of your household that would encourage mental soundness and physical movement. How can you incorporate them into the week? (Examples: family chat night, preparing meal together, cycling, gardening, reading the same title book at the same time and sharing a thought night, etc.)

» Reflect on a time when you made necessary changes (this could have been related to health, finances, relationships, etc.). What steps did you take? What were the results?

NOTES

CHAPTER FOUR
Fuel for the Soul

*Let food be thy medicine
and medicine be thy food.*

HIPPOCRATES, FATHER OF MEDICINE

Besides your mindset, the fuel you will need to reach unthinkable heights is in your refrigerator. A milestone is accomplished when you determine the sources of nutrition that are best for you, and when they should be consumed. In this bid for strength, obstacles leading to transformation are all around. An interruption, or break, in poor eating habits is not an overnight triumph. A lot of the norms you presently embrace come directly from your early experiences with food, and your knowledge of the choices available to you. Early in life we learn to make differentiations in taste so we can discern what pleases the palate as opposed to those things that are unpleasant. However, most of us are not properly educated regarding quality and content of food, or aware of the benefits of certain kinds of foods. Lessons that should help us to respond to questions affecting our health are often missed:

Does the food on my plate represent hues of the rainbow?

- *If I am consuming meat, is it organically raised or processed?*

- Am I hungry, or am I really just dehydrated?

- Am I getting enough calcium?

- The more we question, the more we are likely to discover.

Fuel Your Soul with Meal Prep

One way I remain alert and on the right path to better health is by meal prepping. To meal prep, cook in bulk at the beginning of the week. This practice helps me to save money and use my time wisely. If you are buying every meal, whether fast food or at an indoor eatery, you are probably spending a lot of money. If I know what I am eating for the week, it helps to curb impulsive spending and randomly eating pints of ice cream. Although frequent rewards are acceptable, the money you will save by sticking to a plan is amazing.

Meal prepping allows you to prepare food in many different ways, thereby shaking up the monotony. Try different combinations of food that suit your taste. Although you may have your favorites, eating the same thing every week can get boring. As a remedy, use social media sites like Pinterest and YouTube, and search Google for really cool meal prep plans and food ideas. Cooking can also be therapeutic. It is one of those activities that require active attention. A lot of women I know identify meal prep as a form of self-care.

Benefits of Meal Prep

- *Cost saving*
- *Time saving*
- *Self-care*
- *Accountability*
- *Health*

Savor Your Fuel

While the goal of cooking should be to nourish the entire body, you also want to make sure the foods satisfy the taste buds. Nourishment doesn't have to be flavorless or bland. The most nutritious dishes are often full of flavor. Foods can be flavorful without adding traditional table salts, artery clogging fats, or refined sugar. Some of my favorite organic flavorings are basil, nutmeg, cumin, cayenne pepper, ginseng, rosemary, cilantro, sage, cinnamon, saffron, thyme, and turmeric. The more I experiment with seasonings, the more uses I find for the flavors that delightfully water my taste buds.

Hydrate as a Soul Source

Drinking eight to ten glasses of water per day, before and/or after meals, has been one of the best additions to my healthy eating plan. Oftentimes we are not hungry, but thirsty. Consuming daily recommended amounts of water helps to purify your body of toxins, promote regularity, and give a sense of fullness. A general rule of thumb is to take your weight and divide it by two, take that number and add ounces to that number. Once you start drinking the required amount of water, you just might take a second thought when you are tempted to go back for that second serving of food. Also, it is important to consume between eight and sixteen ounces of a beverage that contains electrolytes. Electrolytes help to stimulate muscles and nerves. In turn, cell function may operate at best levels. Reach out to your doctor and find out how much water you should be drinking daily.

Schedule Your Success

Nutritional consumption on a regular schedule is an important part of developing better habits because your body recalibrates to establish routine schedules. Eating breakfast, lunch, and dinner at a set time may help to promote weight control, lower blood sugar levels, and prevent overeating. For optimal nourishment, regular

50

meals, paired with healthy snacks between meals, aids in supporting a more stabilized metabolism. Some of my patients think that eating one to two times per day will help them to control their weight. They are wrong. You do your body an injustice when you skip meals. A cycle of missing meals is unhealthy and dangerous for many who have health issues. In order to function properly, your body needs a constant flow of proper nutrition.

Energized exercising follows regularly scheduled healthy eating habits. This adds to the energy you need to focus, and supplies the necessary, and essential, vitamins and other nutrients. Foods rich in protein and health-benefiting carbohydrates form the powerhouse to any good workout. Eat foods that are lean and rich in these sources and you will improve the effects of exercise. Pay close attention to carbohydrates that are low on the glycemic index, as they often contain less sugar. In general, notice I say in general, natural foods decrease the likelihood of the dreaded "sugar crash." Most importantly, plan and schedule frequent meals to empower your productivity.

Soul Source Challenges

Anytime you begin a new journey towards health and wellness, you will probably encounter a few challenges along the way. You might have one of those weeks where you exercise vigorously and make all of the right food selections, but to no avail. You opt for lean fish instead of the prime rib at dinner. Your mind may be so made up to follow through that you even skip the chocolate syrup on that coveted "cheat day" ice cream. Sunday rolls around and you rush to the scale to check your weekly progress. And BAM! You have not shed a pound, or you found a pound or two someone else lost that week.

How?

You think to yourself, "How could this be? I did everything right to ensure meeting my goals."

In that moment, you have to decide whether to sidestep the pothole and continue, or to simply give in. I believe your recognition of the challenge at hand is the first step towards real change.

Potholes are expected on any well-traveled road. Expect them to appear. Instead of allowing them to translate to shame and guilt, use them as an opportunity for growth. It is important not to get bogged down with the 'small potholes' along your journey, as you will probably encounter more than one, and with varying levels of difficulty. Regroup, go back to the plan that worked for you in the past, and start fresh. Potholes, or feedback, give us opportunities to make adjustments and realize even greater success.

Oftentimes potholes cease progress. Life happens to all of us, but be prepared and consciously mindful. Permit them to strengthen and sharpen your focus. Alter your beliefs about food and the way you interact with it. Take ownership over the process of healthy eating. Notice I said, "Process of healthy eating." I use this terminology because the best plans evolve as situations evolve. As life, and your lifestyle changes, so should your approach to a health plan. Periodically self-reflect on your progress and your goals. It has been said, "What gets monitored, gets done."

Fit Doc Checkup

Many of our habits, or patterns, are established in childhood. As a youth, what eating choices did you learn that impact the way you interact with food today?

Prep for Success

1. Store left overs in individual serving size containers.

2. Check your calendar and determine meal prep ideas that will fit into your schedules.

3. Purchase portions in single serving packaging, i.e. string cheese, 100 calorie snacks.

4. Check your pantry and refrigerator before each trip to grocery store.

5. Search for different ways to prepare food. Use the Internet and browse magazines.

6. Before shopping, make a list and commit not to veer from it.

7. After washing fresh vegetables and fruits, store individual serving sizes in small baggies. These are great for grabbing when in a pinch for time.

8. Clean the refrigerator weekly. Get rid of left overs that have been around for longer than 3 – 5 days.

9. Plan food and liquid intake.

MONDAY

BREAKFAST

SNACK

LUNCH

SNACK

DINNER

PROTEIN

VEGETABLES

FRUITS

CARBS

OIL/FATS

WATER

TUESDAY

BREAKFAST

SNACK

LUNCH

SNACK

DINNER

PROTEIN

VEGETABLES

FRUITS

CARBS

OIL/FATS

WATER

WEDNESDAY

BREAKFAST

SNACK

LUNCH

SNACK

DINNER

PROTEIN

VEGETABLES

FRUITS

CARBS

OIL/FATS

WATER

THURSDAY

BREAKFAST

SNACK

LUNCH

SNACK

DINNER

PROTEIN

VEGETABLES

FRUITS

CARBS

OIL/FATS

WATER

FRIDAY

BREAKFAST

SNACK

LUNCH

SNACK

DINNER

PROTEIN

VEGETABLES

FRUITS

CARBS

OIL/FATS

WATER

SATURDAY

BREAKFAST

SNACK

LUNCH

SNACK

DINNER

PROTEIN

VEGETABLES

FRUITS

CARBS

OIL/FATS

WATER

60

SUNDAY

BREAKFAST

SNACK

LUNCH

SNACK

DINNER

PROTEIN

VEGETABLES

FRUITS

CARBS

OIL/FATS

WATER

NOTES

CHAPTER FIVE
Move, Move, Move

Schedule an appointment with yourself

According to research, only half of American adults get the recommended amount of at least one hundred fifty minutes of aerobic exercise per week. Some cite busy schedules as the reason for not exercising, but I am a big proponent of "making time." You have it to spare. In fact, you have twenty-four hours, with a series of time commitments to make and honor every day. We frantically scramble to attend to temporal commitments in our daily lives, yet, we fail to consider the ramifications of poor health in carrying out those very same commitments. How you show up in any role you play is in a large way contingent upon your level of health and well-being.

Regular physical activity and exercise impact your health in many ways. You can eat all the fruits and vegetables you want, and sip water all day long. However, if you lead a sedentary lifestyle, you limit your overall health goals.

You have likely heard the phrase, "The best exercise is the exercise you will do." It is not necessary to enroll in a health club or to have access to a track in order to engage in effective exercise. Many of my clients find a way to work up a sweat in their own neighborhoods. The sidewalk can easily serve as a track. You can take the stairs instead of the elevator, or take a short walk during a lunch break. For in home planning, YouTube has millions of instructional exercise presentations. Money for a trainer or gym membership is not always an option for everyone. Search the internet for an exercise plan that starts at your level of comfort. Grab a friend if possible, and remain committed to reaching your fitness goals. Activity that is planned, and intentional, can become a habit. Running is my favorite because it provides great cardiovascular benefits, and I happen to be passionate about the exercise. I have formed a habit of running at least twice per week because it helps to keep my blood flowing and my skin healthy looking. If you are not much of a runner, walking is a great option. Like running, a brisk walk is safe, inexpensive, and easy to do. You can mix up the normal pacing, which potentially burns just as many calories as running.

If starting a new exercise routine seems too daunting, break the workout into smaller, more manageable segments. You can lower the number of sets you complete and add different routines to enhance the training. Try circuit and core training in order to maintain your interest and amplify the results.

Whatever you do, be sure to track your progress and consistently challenge yourself to do more a little at a time. Consult with your doctor to determine the amount of exercise that is right for you, as there are medical conditions that are highly sensitive to certain forms of exercise. It is always a good idea to keep your doctor informed about the type of exercise you are doing. They can share information to help keep you on track and avoid mishaps. Find a program that meets your exercise needs and goals. Remember, aerobic activity will help you burn calories and shed weight. Routines that include working on specific muscle groups can help build strength in the areas you target. Oftentimes people know they want to shed weight, but are doing the wrong exercises to reach their desired outcomes. Consult your physician or a fitness guide who help you to get a better snapshot of what you are trying to accomplish.

As a beginner, or if you are restarting an exercise program at a health club, ask for assistance before using the equipment. The staff should be able to show you how to properly use the exercise machinery. They are knowledgeable in their recommendations for weight lifting limits, and instructing proper posture in the use of each exercise apparatus. This will save you an unnecessary trip to the doctor for an injury that could have been prevented.

Setting appropriate health goals to suit your lifestyle will ultimately come down to you. A lot of the persons I know try to exercise five times per week for thirty to sixty minutes per session. But if that is not feasible for you, start where you can. You can decide on the number of days you can commit to an activity. However, aim for the recommended one hundred fifty minutes of exercise per week. Schedule your training like you do any other important activity in your life. If you do not create a dedicated space just as you do any other responsibility, you will likely treat this necessity as optional.

Develop a new mantra that says, "Training for my health goal is the key to improving my health and wellness."

Exercise and physical activity can improve many aspects of your life. You will feel refreshed, rejuvenated, more confident, healthier, and stronger. For many, exercise decreases grogginess and improves clarity in the brain. As crazy as it may seem, you will likely have more energy in the long run if you expend more energy working out. Regular exercise increases stamina, reduces fatigue, and revs pep into your steps.

A healthy lifestyle that incorporates healthy eating habits and exercise is the key ingredient to the prevention of a range of illnesses. When you exercise, the body produces endorphins, chemicals in the brain that evoke feelings of peace and happiness. This 'feel good' hormone may be an incentive to forming a habit of exercising. While medications help to repair damages, your body's greatest defense is exercise, and the consumption of foods that produce health benefits.

Fit Doc Checkup

1. What are your best physical features? How can you flaunt these features with more intention?

2. Identify physical features you would like to enhance. Design a plan of action.

3. Plan your moves.

WORKOUT PLAN FOR MONDAY

AREA OF TARGET

UPPER BODY - ARMS

TRICEPS

BICEPS

SHOULDERS

CHEST

BACK

MID-SECTION - ABS

OBLIQUE

WAISTLINE

LOWER BODY

HIPS

LEGS

QUADS

BUTTOCKS

CARDIO/AEROBIC

STRETCHES

MEDITATION

RESOURCES/TOOLS
(EXAMPLES: YOUTUBE, DVD, YOGA MAT, ETC.)

WORKOUT PLAN FOR TUESDAY

AREA OF TARGET

UPPER BODY - ARMS

TRICEPS

BICEPS

SHOULDERS

CHEST

BACK

MID-SECTION - ABS

OBLIQUE

WAISTLINE

LOWER BODY

HIPS

LEGS

QUADS

BUTTOCKS

CARDIO/AEROBIC

STRETCHES

MEDITATION

RESOURCES/TOOLS
(EXAMPLES: YOUTUBE, DVD, YOGA MAT, ETC.)

71

WORKOUT PLAN FOR WEDNESDAY

AREA OF TARGET

UPPER BODY - ARMS

TRICEPS

BICEPS

SHOULDERS

CHEST

BACK

MID-SECTION - ABS

OBLIQUE

WAISTLINE

LOWER BODY

HIPS

LEGS

QUADS

BUTTOCKS

CARDIO/AEROBIC

STRETCHES

MEDITATION

RESOURCES/TOOLS
(EXAMPLES: YOUTUBE, DVD, YOGA MAT, ETC.)

72

WORKOUT PLAN FOR THURSDAY

AREA OF TARGET

UPPER BODY - ARMS

TRICEPS

BICEPS

SHOULDERS

CHEST

BACK

MID-SECTION - ABS

OBLIQUE

WAISTLINE

LOWER BODY

HIPS

LEGS

QUADS

BUTTOCKS

CARDIO/AEROBIC

STRETCHES

MEDITATION

RESOURCES/TOOLS
(EXAMPLES: YOUTUBE, DVD, YOGA MAT, ETC.)

73

WORKOUT PLAN FOR FRIDAY

AREA OF TARGET

UPPER BODY - ARMS

TRICEPS

BICEPS

SHOULDERS

CHEST

BACK

MID-SECTION - ABS

OBLIQUE

WAISTLINE

LOWER BODY

HIPS

LEGS

QUADS

BUTTOCKS

CARDIO/AEROBIC

STRETCHES

MEDITATION

RESOURCES/TOOLS
(EXAMPLES: YOUTUBE, DVD, YOGA MAT, ETC.)

74

WORKOUT PLAN FOR SATURDAY

AREA OF TARGET

UPPER BODY - ARMS

TRICEPS

BICEPS

SHOULDERS

CHEST

BACK

MID-SECTION - ABS

OBLIQUE

WAISTLINE

LOWER BODY

HIPS

LEGS

QUADS

BUTTOCKS

CARDIO/AEROBIC

STRETCHES

MEDITATION

RESOURCES/TOOLS
(EXAMPLES: YOUTUBE, DVD, YOGA MAT, ETC.)

WORKOUT PLAN FOR SUNDAY

AREA OF TARGET

UPPER BODY - ARMS

TRICEPS

BICEPS

SHOULDERS

CHEST

BACK

MID-SECTION - ABS

OBLIQUE

WAISTLINE

LOWER BODY

HIPS

LEGS

QUADS

BUTTOCKS

CARDIO/AEROBIC

STRETCHES

MEDITATION

RESOURCES/TOOLS
(EXAMPLES: YOUTUBE, DVD, YOGA MAT, ETC.)

NOTES

NOTES

CHAPTER SIX
The Cool Down

"If you neglect to recharge a battery, it dies. And if you run full-speed ahead without stopping for water, you lose momentum to finish the race."

OPRAH WINFREY

Your Life is Your Hands

I imagine you are a superwoman...with the capability to wake up at ungodly hours of the morning, cook breakfast, dress your kids (maybe your spouse too), work eight to ten, pick up the kids from school, make dinner, and everything else under the sun. During the span of a single day you will wear many hats: wife, mother, employee, employer, caretaker, motivator, friend, and perhaps serve in many other roles. The cape never comes off. And, like most superheroes, you will not always get the glory you deserve.

Your efforts to meet the needs of everyone else before your own will run you ragged if you do not set boundaries. Thus, learning to take care of oneself may be a new concept for many of us. We spend so much of our days managing the well-being of other people that we neglect the most important person ourselves. However, it is important to remember, you are responsible for the vessel you carry. Anything and everything that will manifest in your life will be as a result of the choices you make form

80

moment to moment. As much as you may be encouraged to make healthy food selections and to exercise consistently, this book is a self-care guide on how to live a life that is fulfilling to the core.

Self-care is recognizing your needs and being intentional about meeting them in ways that are both beneficial and health promoting. It is about taking the time to treat yourself with the utmost love, respect, and care you deserve. The same energy that you invest into making sure that others are the best of the best, should be invested into yourself. If needs be, discard the feelings of shame and guilt in order to replenish the cups you fill so freely for others. Self-care is not selfish it is wellness at its finest.

It's Time to Fully Engage

As a doctor, I am often under unbelievable pressure to perform at my best. More often than not, I do not take the time to have a sit-down lunch... without interruptions. Typically, you can find me eating my lunch while answering telephone calls. My staff works really hard as well. We are all performing at very high levels, with narrow pauses for breathers. For the past few years, I have been addressing our need to recharge. Although there are many ways to approach this concept, as an initiative to relaxing during the work day, I employ a masseuse into the office twice per week. My patients, staff and I have benefited greatly from this therapeutic practice, and aspire to continue as part of our tradition.

Massages are an excellent way to relieve anxiety, stress, and improve your overall mood. Most people notice an immediate shift in spirit after a massage. Since I exercise quite often, massages are an important part of my regiment in the prevention of muscle overuse. A really good massage therapy session may prove pivotal in the alleviation of tension in your muscles. Less muscle tension reduces certain injuries, thereby creating a measure of calm in your life.

Self-care is about taking extra strides to ensure your body and mind perform optimally. Most of us will admit we could use more rest and reset in our lives. More often than not, I shut down my phone and detach from the social media world so I can be present and fully engage with myself. Quiet moments of solitude is necessary. I love to spend time in complete stillness, allowing my mind to recuperate and set new coordinates. In this current era of checking social media every minute and every hour, your inner GPS can easily be derailed.

It Gets Personal

My signature red lipstick is not complete without a well-coordinated pedicure. A visit to the nail salon for a manicure and pedicure has a way of soothing your precious limbs. Pampering and beautification are surefire ways to invest in yourself. Although I prefer to let someone else take care of my hands and feet, the act of giving to yourself is refreshing as well. Pampering your own nails and caring for your feet are two great ways to completely zone out and hone in on self.

Taking care of your crown is a must for any self-care regimen. The inner diva is noticeable when a woman has a fresh "do." Women have told me that they feel better after a visit to the hair salon. A great hairstyle, I believe, has the power to unleash inner confidence that exudes from one's pores and radiates to others. When I make it a point to visit my stylist weekly, it is a way for me to ensure that my physical appearance is nurtured, so that I am presenting my best self both to me and to the world.

An overlooked opportunity for self-care can be found in the way we connect with others. As humans, we are relational beings. Breaks from norms and life's routines are essential sources of inspiration and energy. Make it a point to check-in with people you have not seen in a while. It is important that we maintain relationships that nourish our souls. As much as this journey is about maintaining the joy of self, our lessons in this race must be transferred and heard by others.

Acknowledge life's simple pleasures that bring you joy. I love hanging out on the beach whether it is hot or cold. The water is calming in and of itself, but add the crashing waves and the beaming sun and I am transported to a faraway land. The outdoors, and becoming one with the sun, is one of the ways I choose to affirm my existence. When I am outside I feel free and connected to something larger than myself. It allows me to reflect on the smallness of my mission and the enormity of the possibilities for impacting others. I am inspired to become who I am intended to be, more and more, and day by day. Self-care reflects an expression of self on a grand scale.

Moment by moment, honor the trail you were created to blaze. The ultimate goal of this lifestyle enhancement is love of self, and it is commanded in order for us to truly care for others.

I Corinthians 6:19 reminds us, "Or do you not know that your body is the temple of the Holy Spirit who is in you, whom you have from God, and you are not your own?" By all accounts, self-love is a form of honoring the body and the Spirit within. To feel good, and to be guided, motivated, affirmed, and ultimately purposeful are keys to being your best self. Please be kind to yourself as you continue to run this race. I urge you to inspire others while training alongside them, or forge ahead on a road that eventually leads to health, wellness, and fitness. As the saying goes, "When you look good, you feel good." However, I like to say "When you feel good, you look good."

Fit Doc Checkup

» How do you currently focus on your needs? Design a self-care plan that honors who you are and who you are becoming.

» Engage with Dr. Michele on Twitter @FitDocMicheleR. Tweet your top 3 action steps you will commit to take. Use hashtag #FitDoc and Dr. Michele will correspond with you.

NOTES

RESOURCES
My Top 5 Health and Wellness Apps Right Now

Sworkit – if you are not a fan of going to the gym, this may be a great alternative. It provides customized workout plans that can be done on the go.

7 Minute Workout – Sometimes we do not have that much time to work out. However, if you invest a few minutes per day in your health and wellness, you are putting yourself in a better position than if you do nothing.

Ziongo – I love the mission of this company. Their mission is to reduce chronic disease by examining the health of what you eat. They work with health professionals to decide the healthiest food options available whether you are at work, home, or eating out.

Rise – Nutrition coaches can be really expensive. The Rise app gives you access to a nutrition coach at a really low price from the comfort of your phone. For less than $2 a day, you can be well on your way to meeting your fitness goals.

Charity Miles- Sometimes we need to do something that is bigger than ourselves. Charity Miles is the app for you if you are a runner and looking to give to a noble cause. Various charities have agreed to donate money to a special cause, all in exchange for your miles.

Acknowledgments

God has blessed me with a circle of so many amazing people and experiences over my lifetime. Each of you have been a part of FitDoc's journey that has continued to shape me to be the person that I am today.

Growing up, my grandparents would always tell us that their goal in life was to have each generation strive to be better than the generation before them. I am grateful that my last grandparent lived long enough to see me become a physician and to open up my own office with two locations.

Thank you to my husband, Scott, whose unwavering support means the world to me and our two sons.

My circle also includes my parents, mother-in-law, siblings, siblings-in-love, family, friends and MS Family Medicine Health Care, P.C. staff and patients.

I would also like to thank the Congregational Church of South Hempstead, the NAACP, National Coalition of 100 Black Women Long Island Chapter, Inc., Alpha Kappa Alpha Sorority, Inc., Black Girls Run (especially the past and present ambassadors) and Merrick Bicycles Triathlon Team.

The outline of my book was completed over two years but I would like to thank Linda Dunn for introducing me to Dr. Larthenia Howard, my Book Coach at the Odyssey Network Business Retreat. Through this process, Dr. Larthenia and I have truly formed a lasting bond.

Thank you to my Brand Manager, Daunte Henderson, for keeping me on task especially after I have had a long day in the office.

Randi, Lindsay and Jeff, thank you for knowing what looks best on me so that I can always look amazing.

Thank you Tamara for keeping my makeup flawless! You are the best!

Phil, you are an amazing hair stylist and I love your personality and skills.

I would like to thank my team of supporters for keeping me healthy and strong: Dr. Smith, Dr. Ohri, Dr. Achampong, Dr. Jen, Dr. Marlissa, and Masseuse, Kim Jackson

A huge thank you to Coach Jaclyn Fahey and Coach Lancelot Theobold for keeping me on track with training. I'm grateful for your support.

Fit Doc Programs and Services

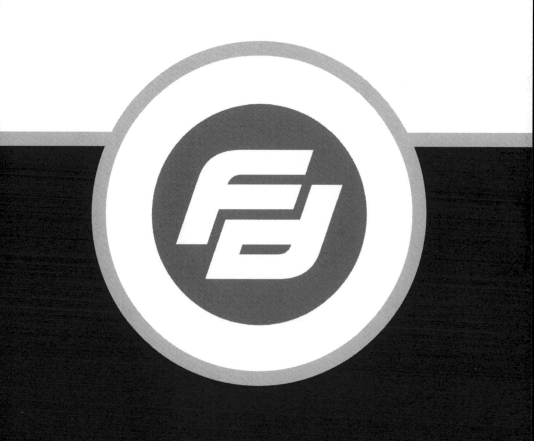

Services and Programs

Keynote Address

Health and Wellness Speech and Lecture

Private and Group Coaching

Panel Guest Speaker

Contact Dr. Michele at www.fitdoc.com

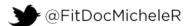 @FitDocMicheleR

#FitDoc

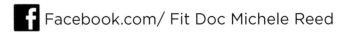 Facebook.com/ Fit Doc Michele Reed

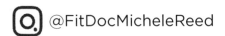 @FitDocMicheleReed

94

About the Author

Dr. Michele Claudette Reed (Fit Doc) is a practicing Board Certified Family Medicine Physician and the owner and Medical Director of MS Family Medicine Health Care, P.C., a holistic practice that serves two locations in Rosedale Queens and Garden City, New York. Dr. Reed also serves as the School District Physician for the Malverne and Roosevelt School Districts in Nassau County, NY. Dr. Reed remains committed to serving her community and also serves as the community the Medical Director for The Congregational Church of South Hempstead.

From an early age, Dr. Reed had aspirations of becoming a doctor and has dedicated her life to serving her community and working as an advocate for overall wellness and the prevention of chronic diseases.

Dr. Reed is extremely passionate about living her best life and motivating her patients and peers to join her on this journey. Dr. Reed is deeply rooted in the fabric of the community where she spearheads health initiatives for the numerous organizations where she serves including, National Coalition of 100 Black Women, Long Island Chapter. She is a member of Alpha Kappa Alpha Sorority, Incorporated, NAACP- Lakeview Chapter (Life Member), Black Girls Run (Long Island), a board member of the Queens Chapter of the American Academy of Family Physicians, an Adjunct Clinical Assistant Professor at New York Medical College and New York College of Osteopathic Medicine, an Executive Board member of the New York College of Osteopathic Medicine Alumni Association, a Fellow of the American Board of Family Medicine.

In the spring of 2014, Dr. Reed was appointed Fellow to the Office of the National Coordinator for Health IT under the Department of Health and Human Services.

Dr. Reed is a recipient of numerous awards and accolades from the local and national community. One of Dr. Reed's greatest accomplishments was completing The NYC Marathon in the fall of 2015. Since then she completed the Chicago Marathon (Oct 2016) and has challenged herself to run half-marathons in all 50 states.

Most recently, Dr. Reed and her husband, Scott Kershaw, Esq. entered a joint venture managing NX Generation Athletics in Westbury, NY. The synergy of medicine and fitness allows Dr. Reed to provide a holistic experience for patients allowing them to incorporate training and exercise into their wellness program.

Dr. Reed and her work have been featured on the Rachael Ray Show with Dr. Ian Smith and Sunny Anderson of the Food Network, Government Technology Today Magazine, Newsday, Verizon Fios News 1 "Push Pause", The New York Daily News, Ebony Magazine, Essence Magazine, Heart and Soul Magazine, and BlackDoctors.org. Additionally, Dr. Reed is a weekly contributor to Late Night Parents with Ted Hicks and Rich Valdez.

Dr. Reed received her undergraduate degree from the State University of New York at Stony Brook and her medical degree from the New York College of Osteopathic Medicine. She is a Long Island native where she lives with her with her husband and twin sons.

34631359R00068

Made in the USA
Middletown, DE
01 February 2019